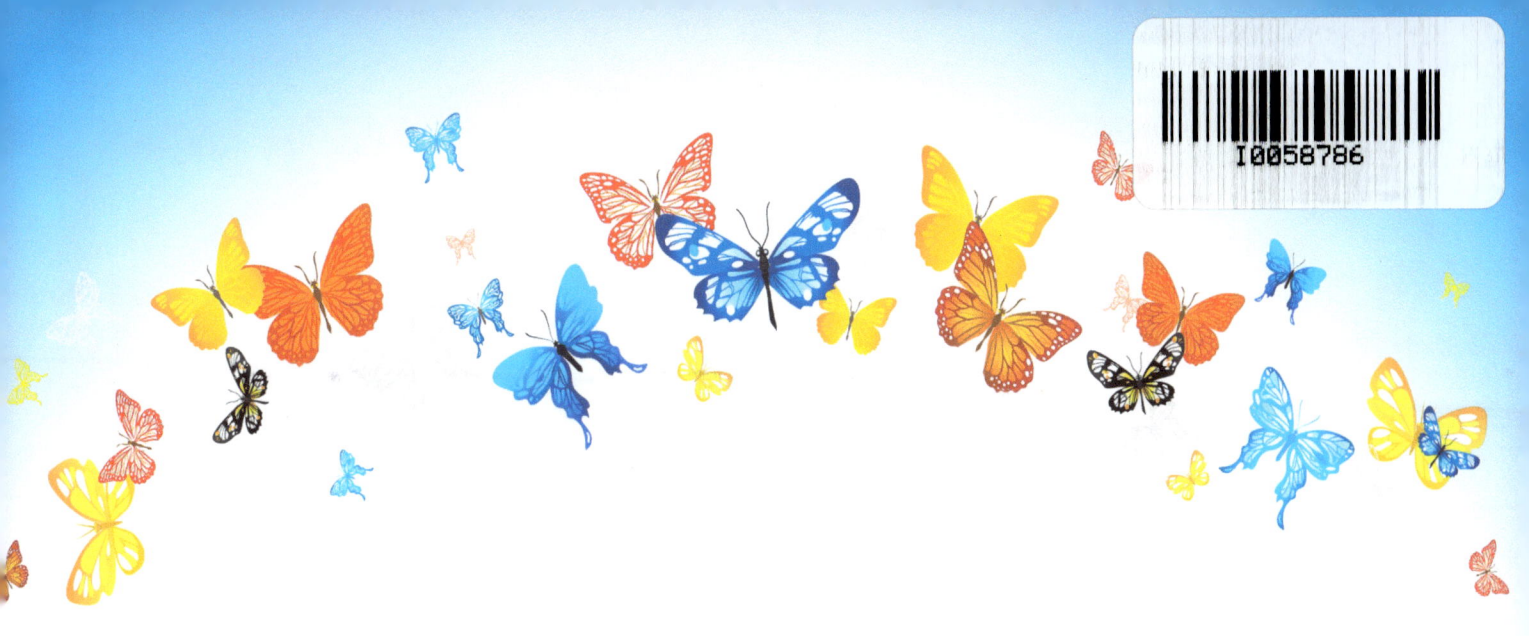

"Amazing Kids' Stories by a Kid"

Part Two

By Anoushka Parag Mahajan

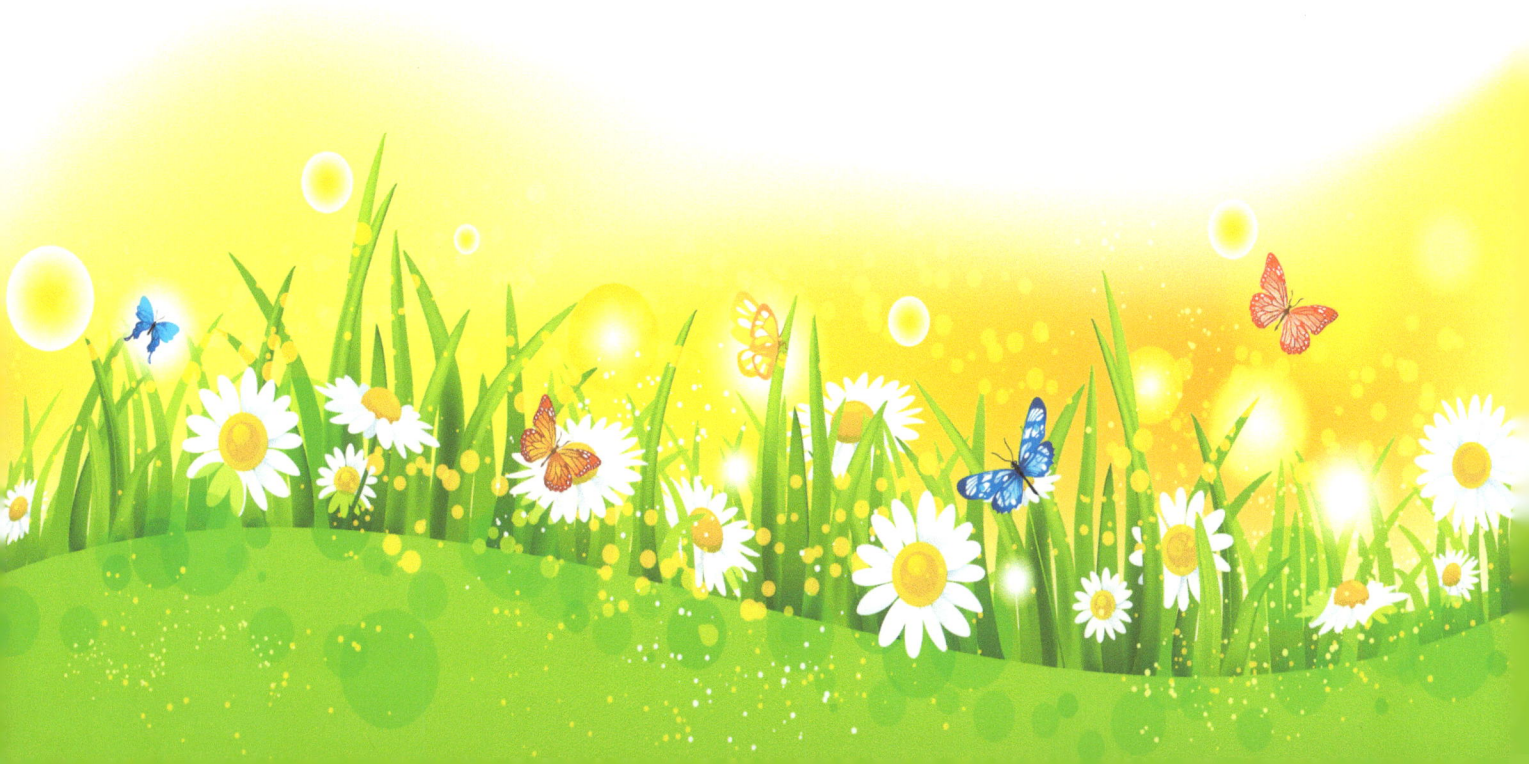

"Amazing Kids' Stories by a Kid - Part 2" Written and Published by Anoushka Parag Mahajan, B3/102, Plot No. 239, RDP-6, Kesar CHS, Charkop Market, Charkop, Mumbai, India - 400067

www.MedMantra.com/apm

© 2018 Anoushka Parag Mahajan

Hardcover Print Book ISBN: 978-93-5281-773-3

Paperback Print Book ISBN: 978-93-5281-725-2

E-book ISBN: 978-93-5281-643-9

CONTENTS

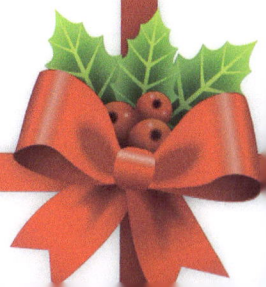

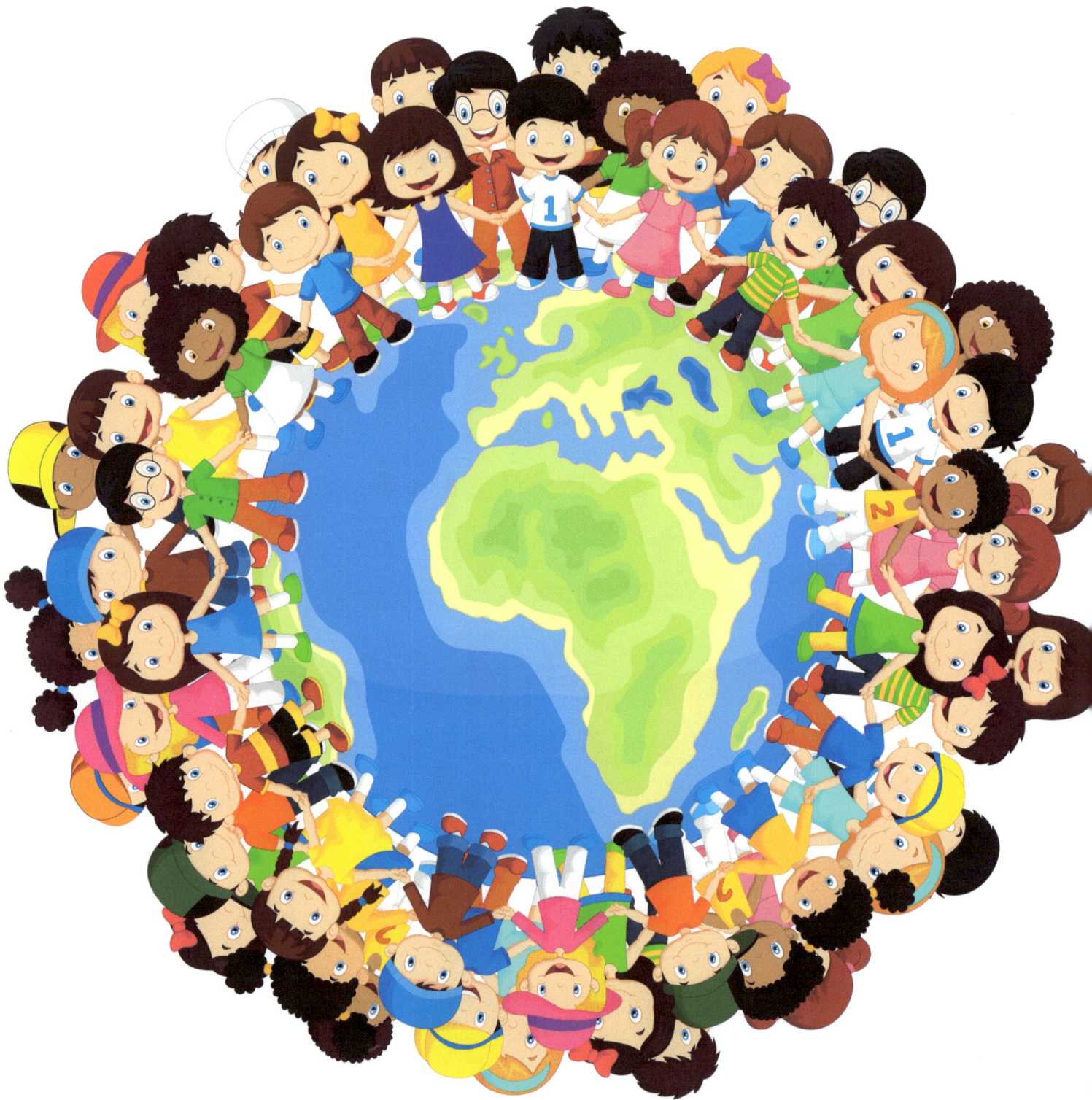

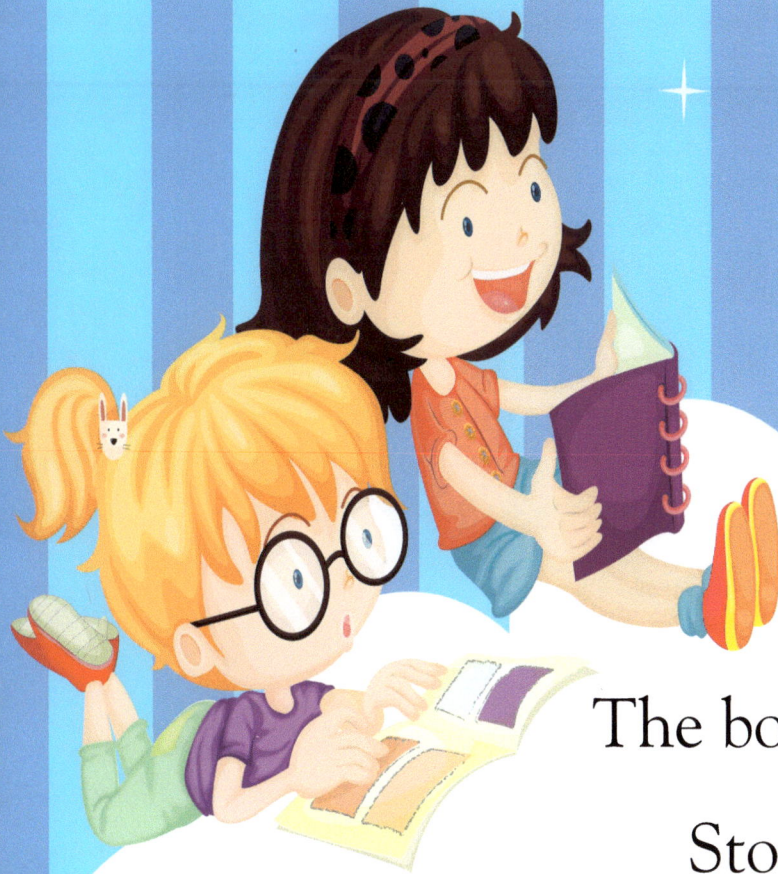

The book 'Amazing Kids' Stories by a Kid' is

a gift from me to all the young kids on

my tenth birthday.

Anoushka Mahajan

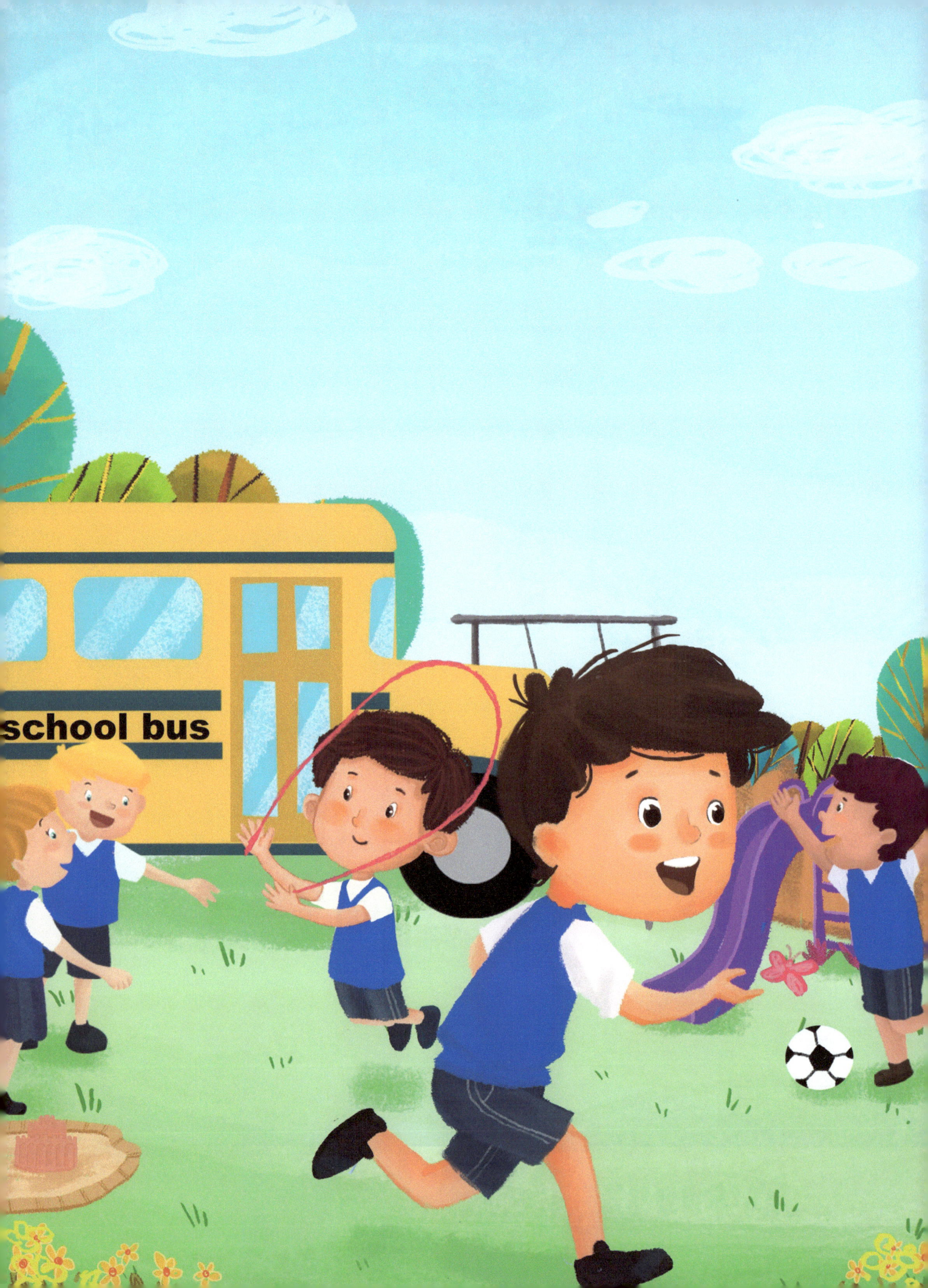

school bus

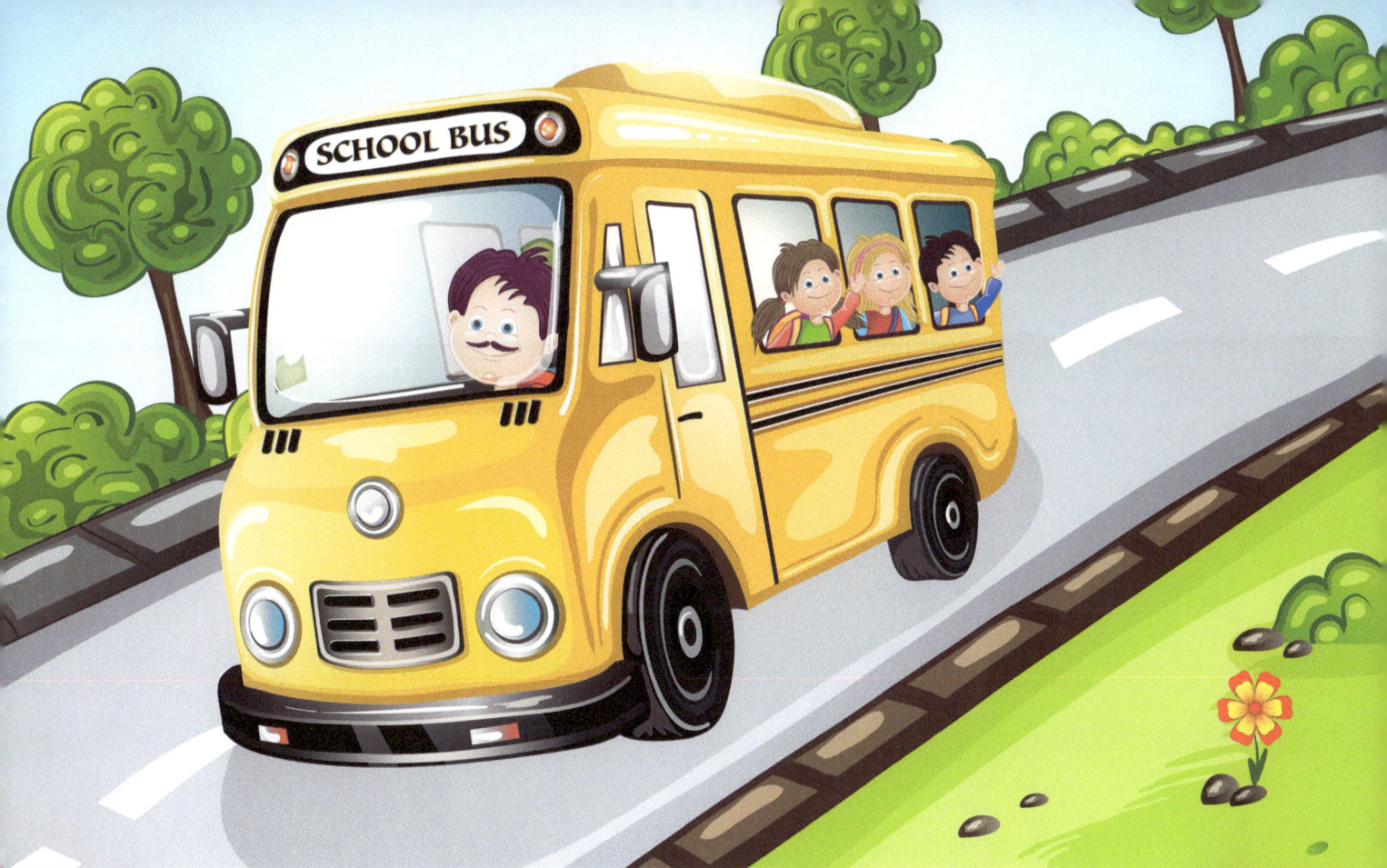

BUMBA GETS LOST WHILE ON HIS SCHOOL PICNIC

Bumba was a very adventurous little boy.

When his class teacher said that the children would be taken on a picnic soon, he was very excited.

He kept asking his mom and dad when it was going to be the picnic day.

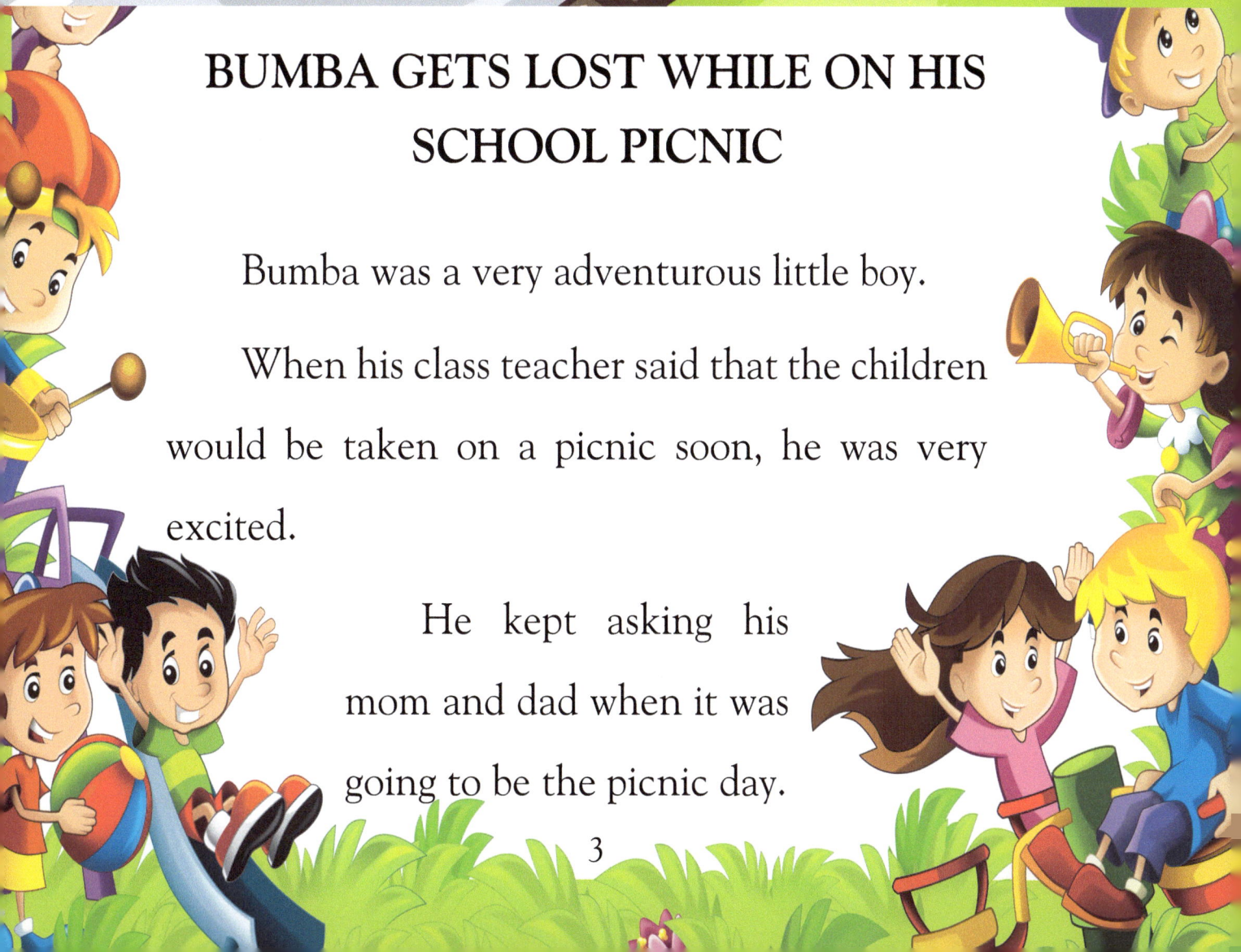

He asked so many times, that his mom said, "Stop asking the same question hundred times!"

He said, "Okay."

But he still asked the same question many times.

A few days later, his mom said, "Bumba, tomorrow you will be going on your school picnic, so sleep early tonight."

And so Bumba went to sleep early. In his sleep, he dreamed of all the fun things he could do on his school picnic tomorrow. He was so happy that he was laughing in his sleep.

It dawned to the day of the picnic…

Bumba sprang out of bed excitedly and got ready all by himself.

Then he got into the bus and went to school.

Once he reached school, he got into another bus along with all the other children to go on the picnic. Along the way, they sang songs and clapped hands.

Finally, they reached the park where they were going to have their picnic.

At the park, Bumba played with his friends. He played and he played, he had a lot of fun.

The teacher said to the children, "Don't go anywhere alone. Stay close to each other."

All the children listened to the teacher and stayed close to one another.

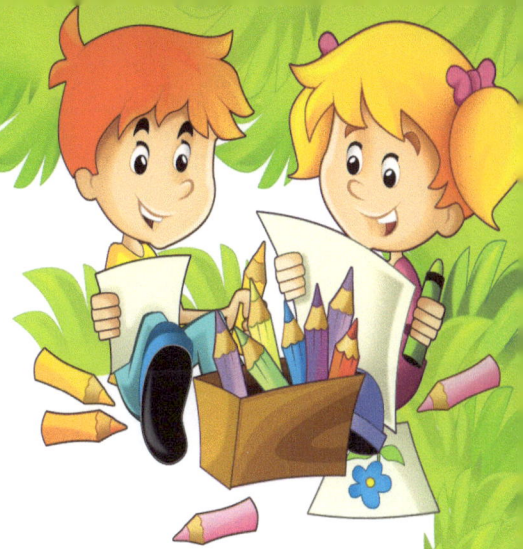

But while he was playing, Bumba was having so much fun that he forgot what his teacher said. He ran everywhere all alone, and after some time, he got lost.

He searched and searched, but he couldn't find the other children.

Soon, the other children were going back home. Bumba's teacher did not know that Bumba had gotten lost. They left without him.

When Bumba noticed that the bus and the other children were nowhere to be seen, he got very scared and he started to cry.

But there was no one to help him.

Moral: listen to your teacher and never forget what she or he says.

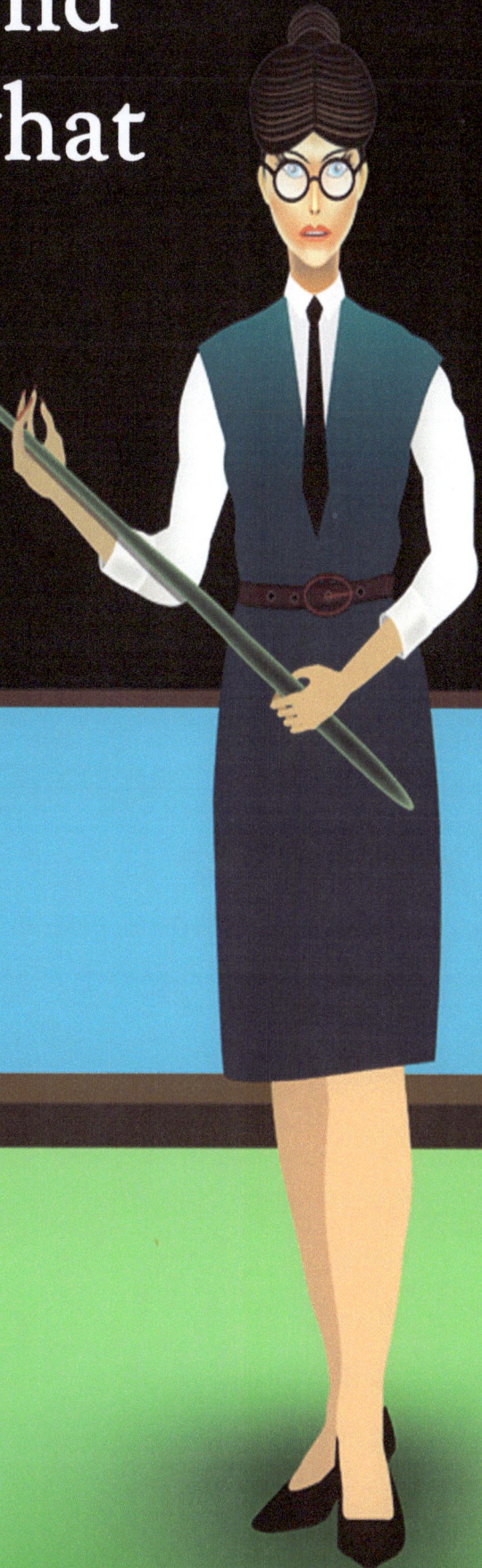

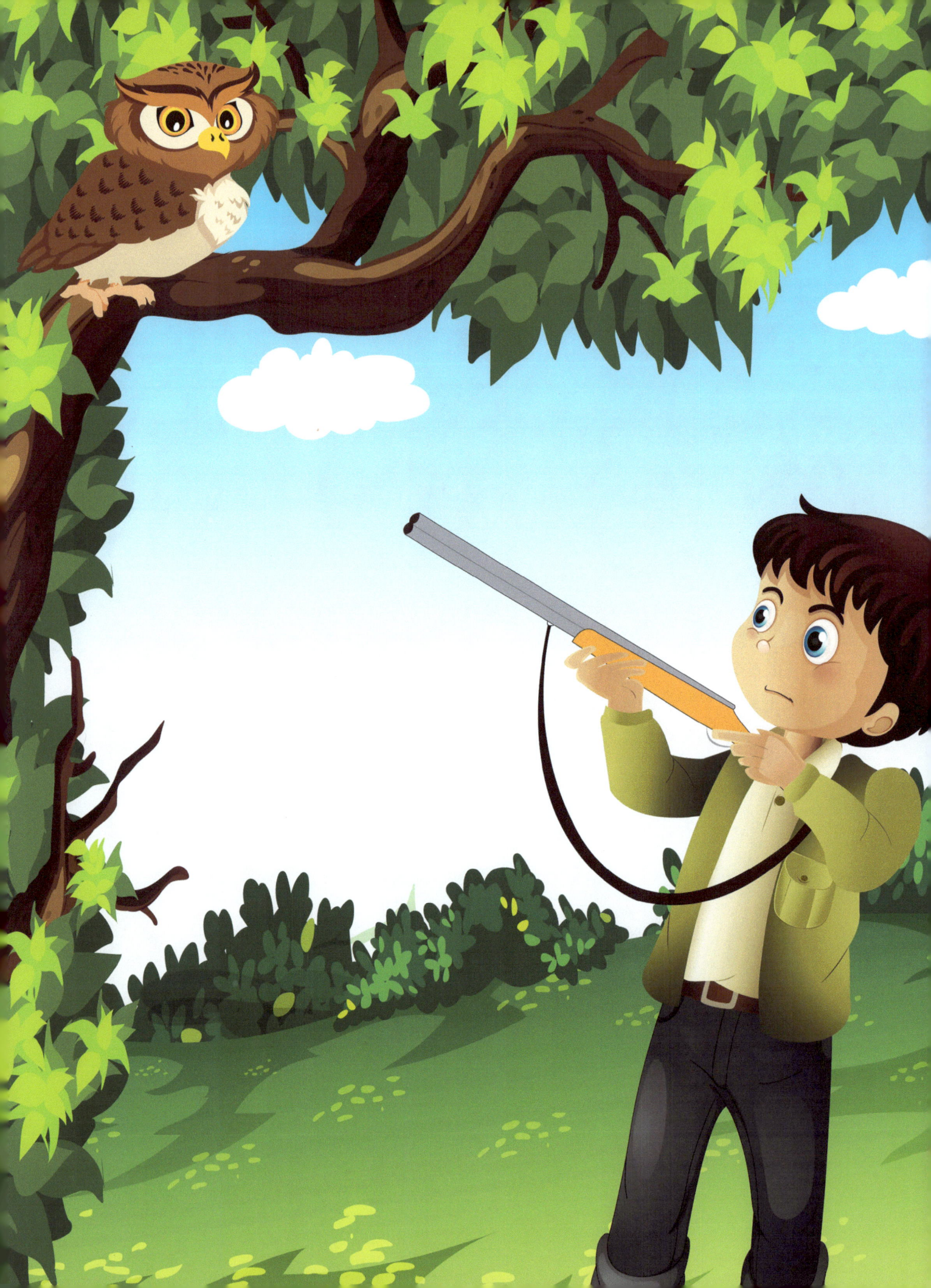

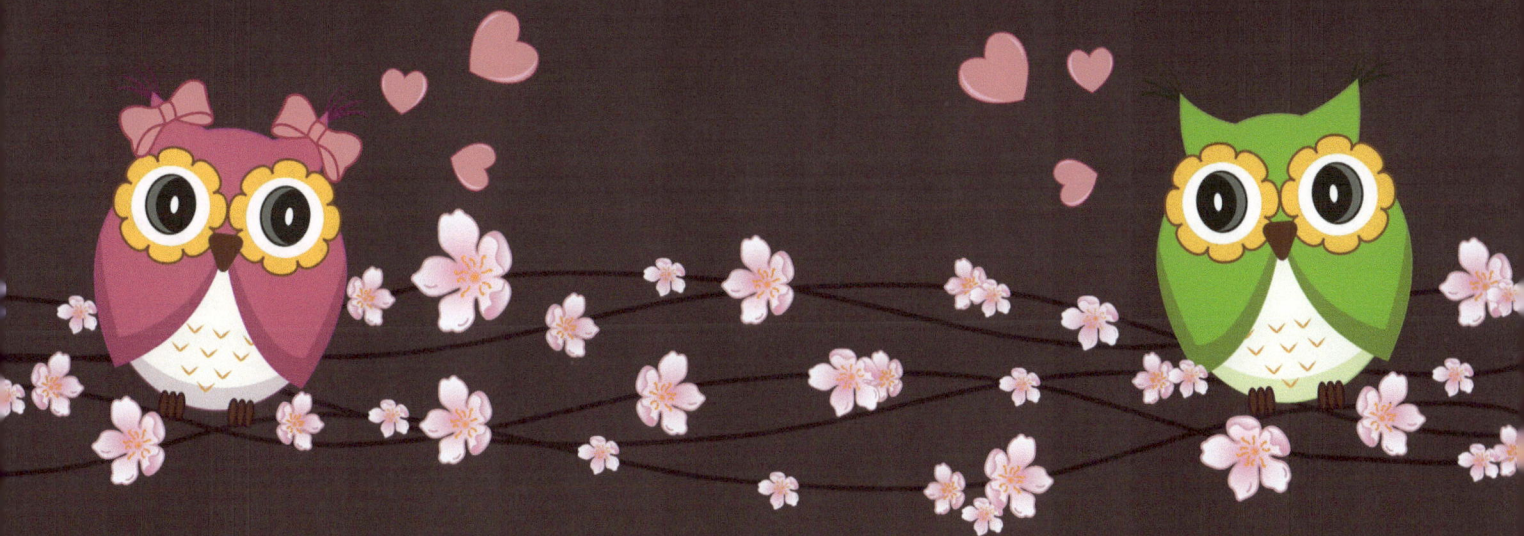

THE BOY AND THE OWL

Once upon a time, there was a very naughty little boy. He lived with his mother, father, sister, and brother.

His father was a police officer, and his mother was a teacher.

One day, his mother and father went to work as usual, and the boy's brother and sister were studying.

The boy sneaked into his parent's room and took his father's gun. Without making any noise, he went out of his home.

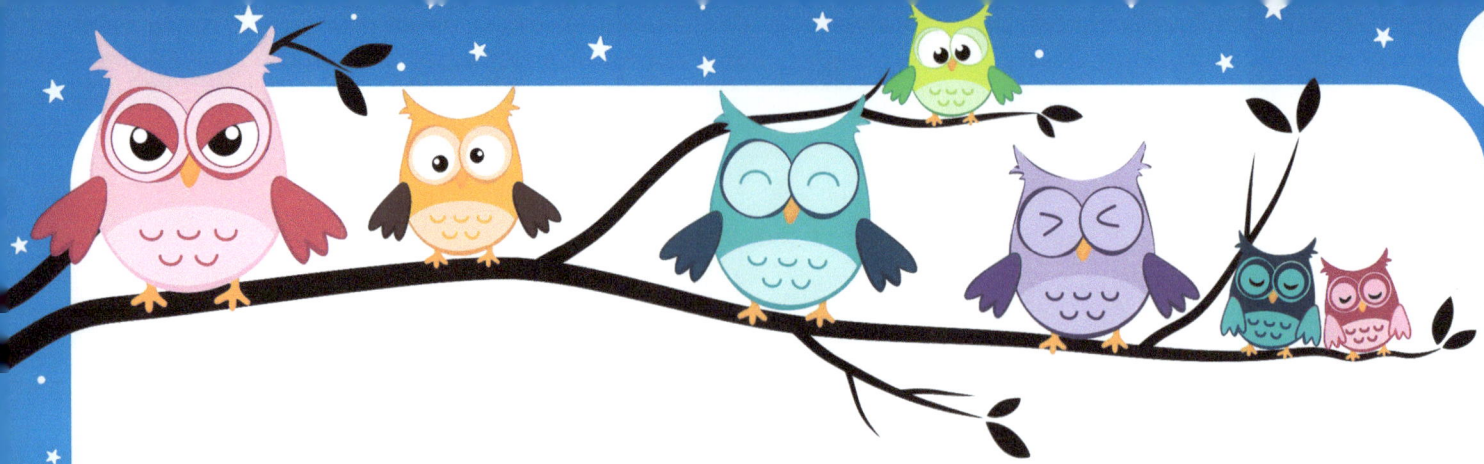

He walked towards the woods, and there he saw an owl perched on a tree top. He thought, 'I must shoot down this owl.'

So, he began to shoot at the owl. But he missed the first shot. A man who was nearby heard the sound of the gunshot and then he saw the boy shooting at the owl.

The man had three pencils with him. He started to throw the pencils at the boy.

The boy got hurt. He yelled at the man, "Why are you beating me?"

The man said, "Then why are you shooting at the owl?"

The boy replied, "So, what if I want to shoot the owl? I can do as I want!"

The man said, "So what if I want to beat you? I can do what I want!"

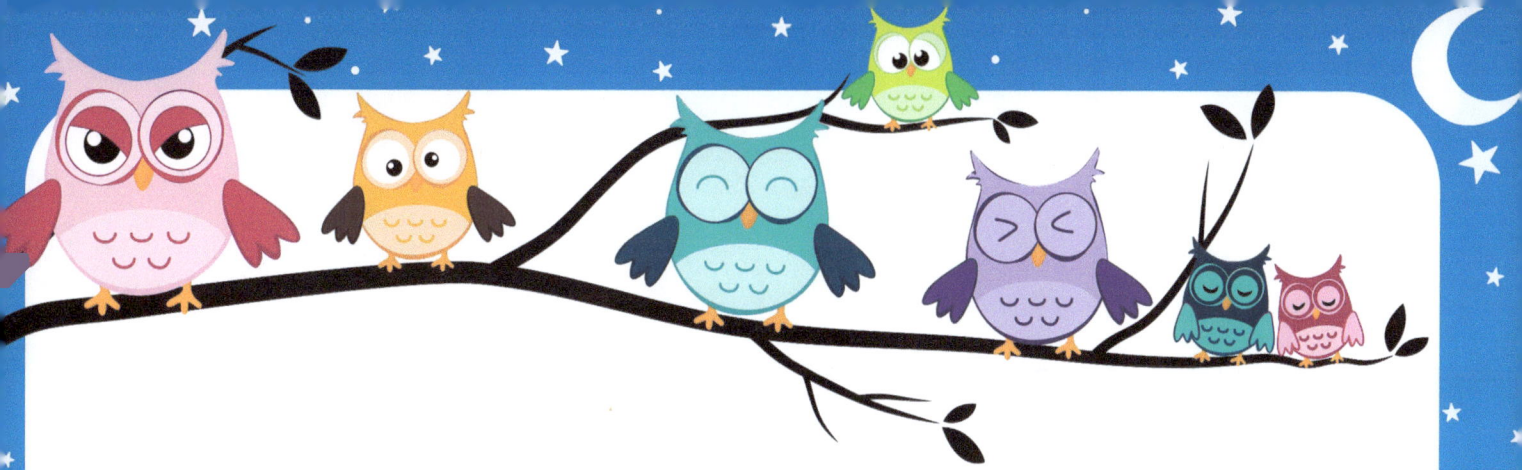

But the boy didn't listen to the man. The man was disappointed by the boy's actions. The man left, since he had some work to do.

So, the boy continued to shoot at the owl.

Just then, his mother and father returned home. They saw that the boy was shooting at the owl.

They told him, "Don't do it. Hurting animals is wrong. They feel pain just the way humans do."

The boy looked down and apologized. He said, "Yes, when the man threw pencils at me, it hurt. So, the same way, if I shoot at the owl it will hurt the owl. Now I understand that animals are our friends."

His mother and father took the boy home with them.

Moral: Animals and birds are our friends. So, don't kill them, protect them.

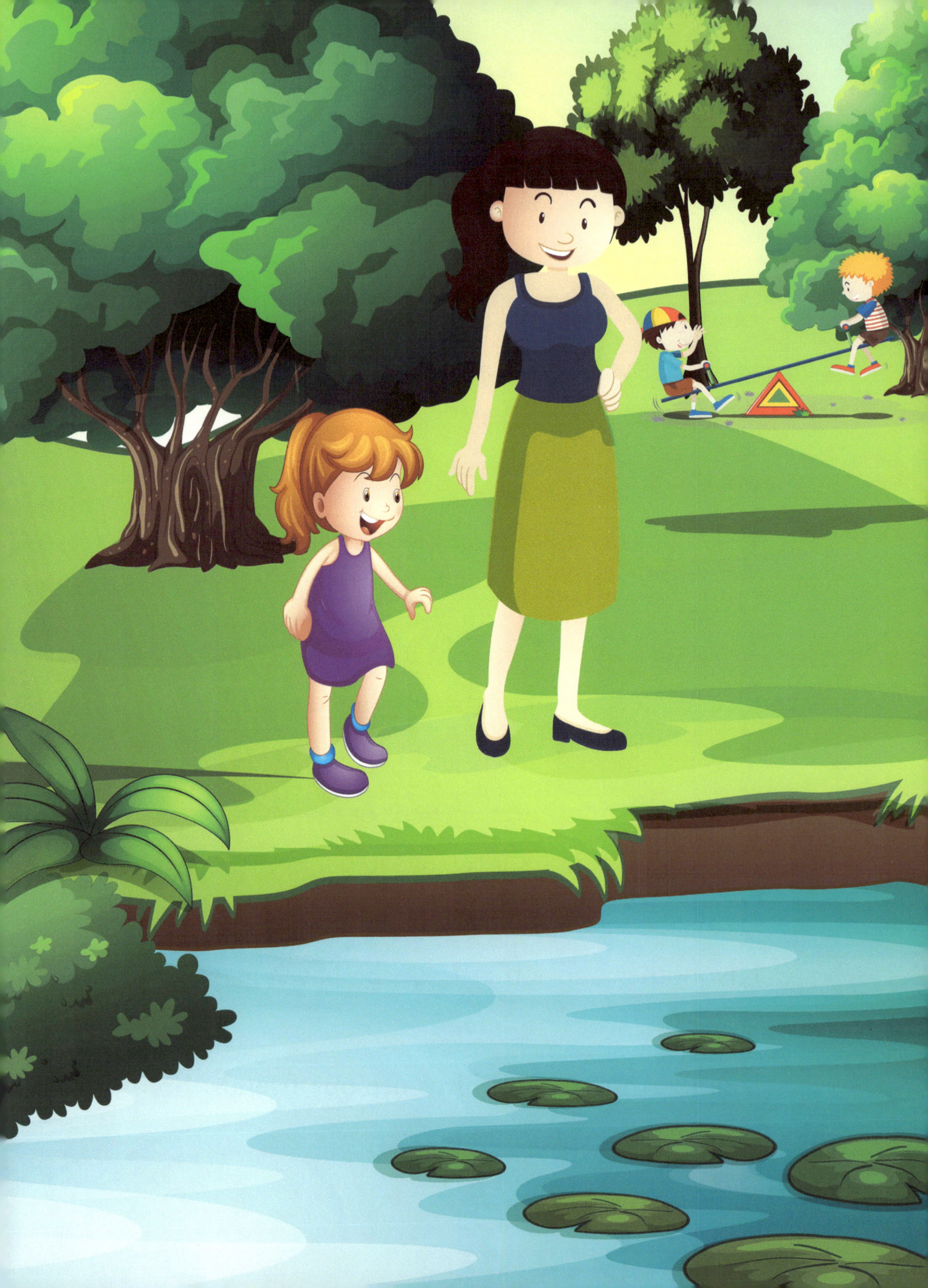

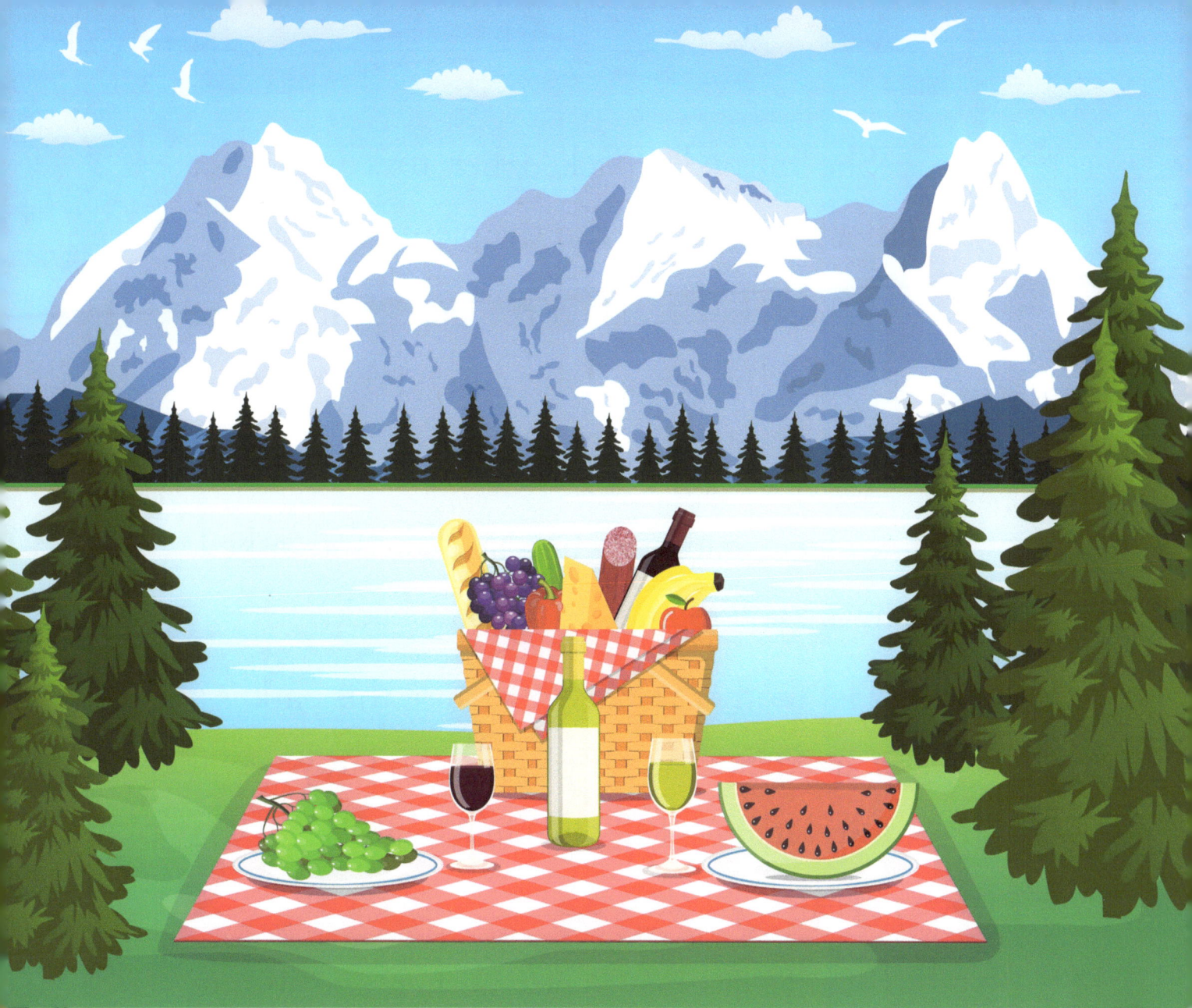

SUMIYA'S PICNIC WITH HER FAMILY

"It's picnic time!" Sumiya's mother said on a Saturday morning.

Little Sumiya was excited and happy to hear this. She loved to go on picnics with her mother and father.

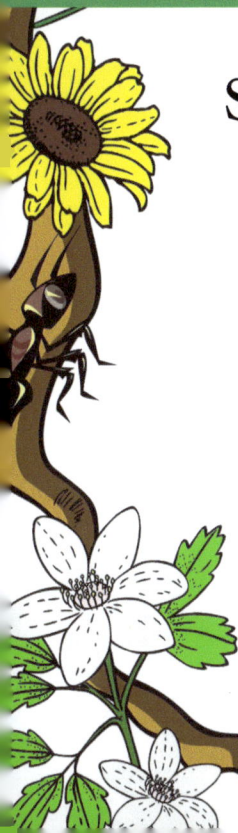

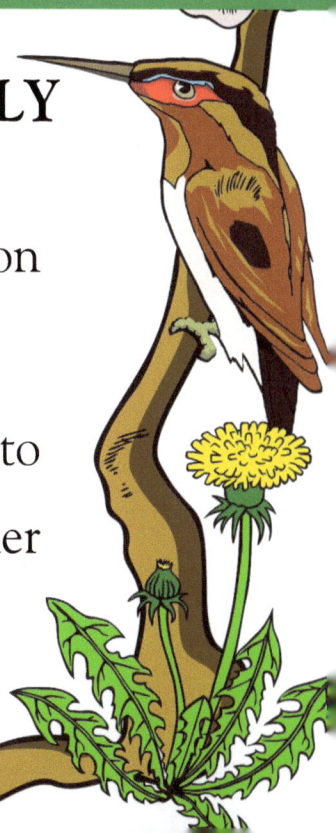

She hurriedly packed her toys while her mother packed food into the picnic basket.

When they reached the park, Sumiya got down from the car and ran around the park.

Her mother yelled, "Come back, Sumiya!"

Sumiya came to her mother and asked, "Why are you telling me to come back?"

Her mother replied, "Because this park is a very large place, and if you run too far, you will get lost. First, we will have lunch, and then you can play."

Sumiya listened to her mother, and she ate the food very quickly.

Then she told her mother, "Let's go to play, mother."

Her mother replied, "Okay, let's go."

Sumiya played in the park while her mother watched.

Suddenly, Sumiya noticed a small pond by the side of the park. She asked her mother whether they could swim in the water.

Her mother replied, "No, we did not bring our swim suits."

Just then, her father called out to her mother. Her mother told her, "I will come back in a little while."

Sumiya said, "Okay, mother."

Her mother went to her father.

Sumiya thought, 'let me go in the water, I will come back before mother comes.'

She went into the water and swam around happily. After some time, she got bored. She wanted to come out, but she did not know from where she could get out because some places were deep.

She couldn't find a shallow area so she could get out.

She began to cry.

Then, one man heard her cries and asked her, "What happened?"

She told him, "I don't know from where to come out of this pond."

The man showed her the shallow area of the pond, and he helped her out of the water.

The next moment, Sumiya's mother arrived. Sumiya ran to her mother.

Her mother asked, "Where have you been? Why are your clothes drenched?"

Sumiya replied, "I went into the water but did not know from where to come out. Then one uncle came and helped me to come out of the water."

Her mother advised her, "You should never go anywhere alone. You must always go with father and me."

Moral: Never go anywhere alone, go with your parents.

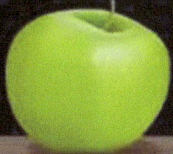

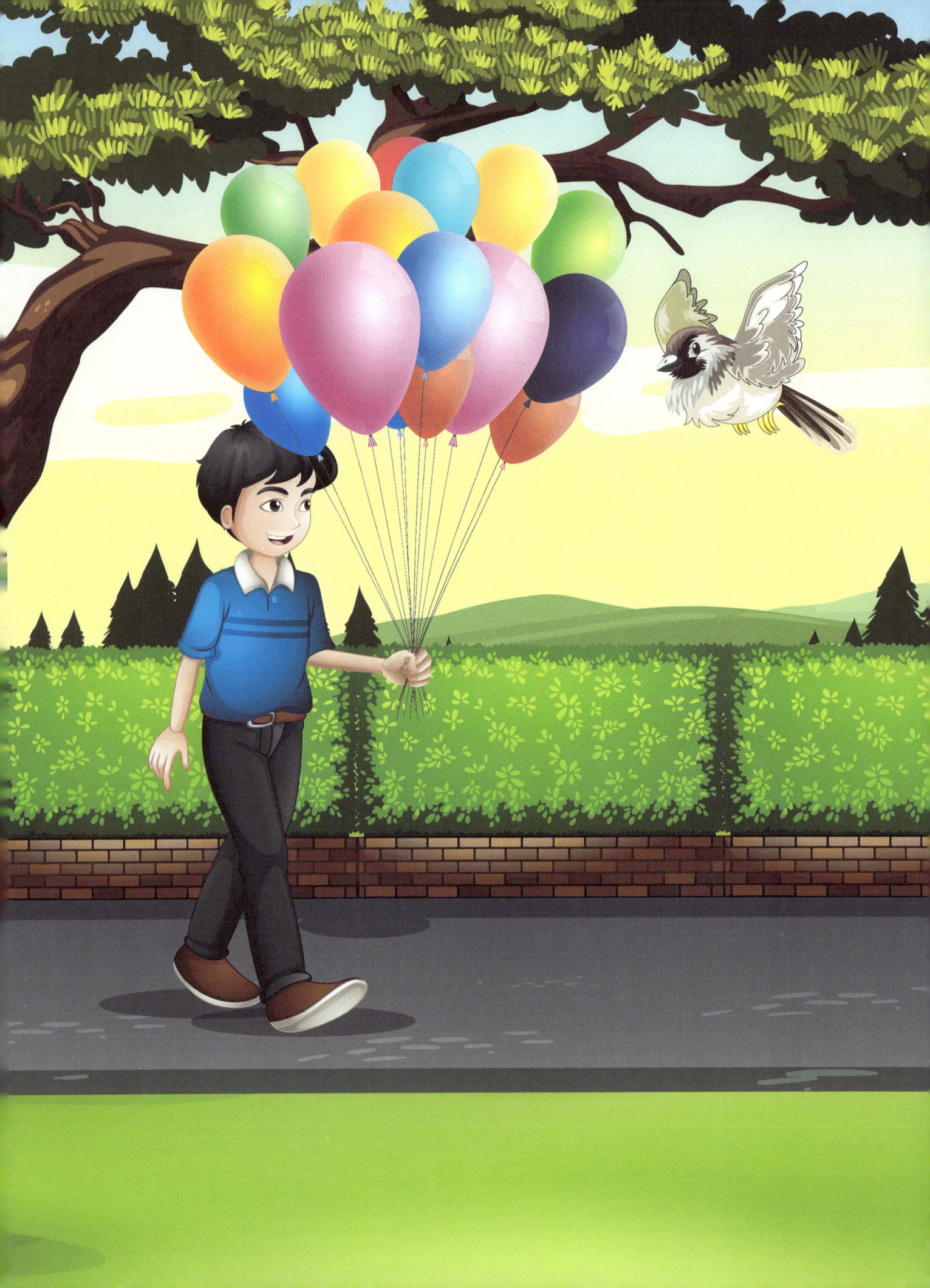

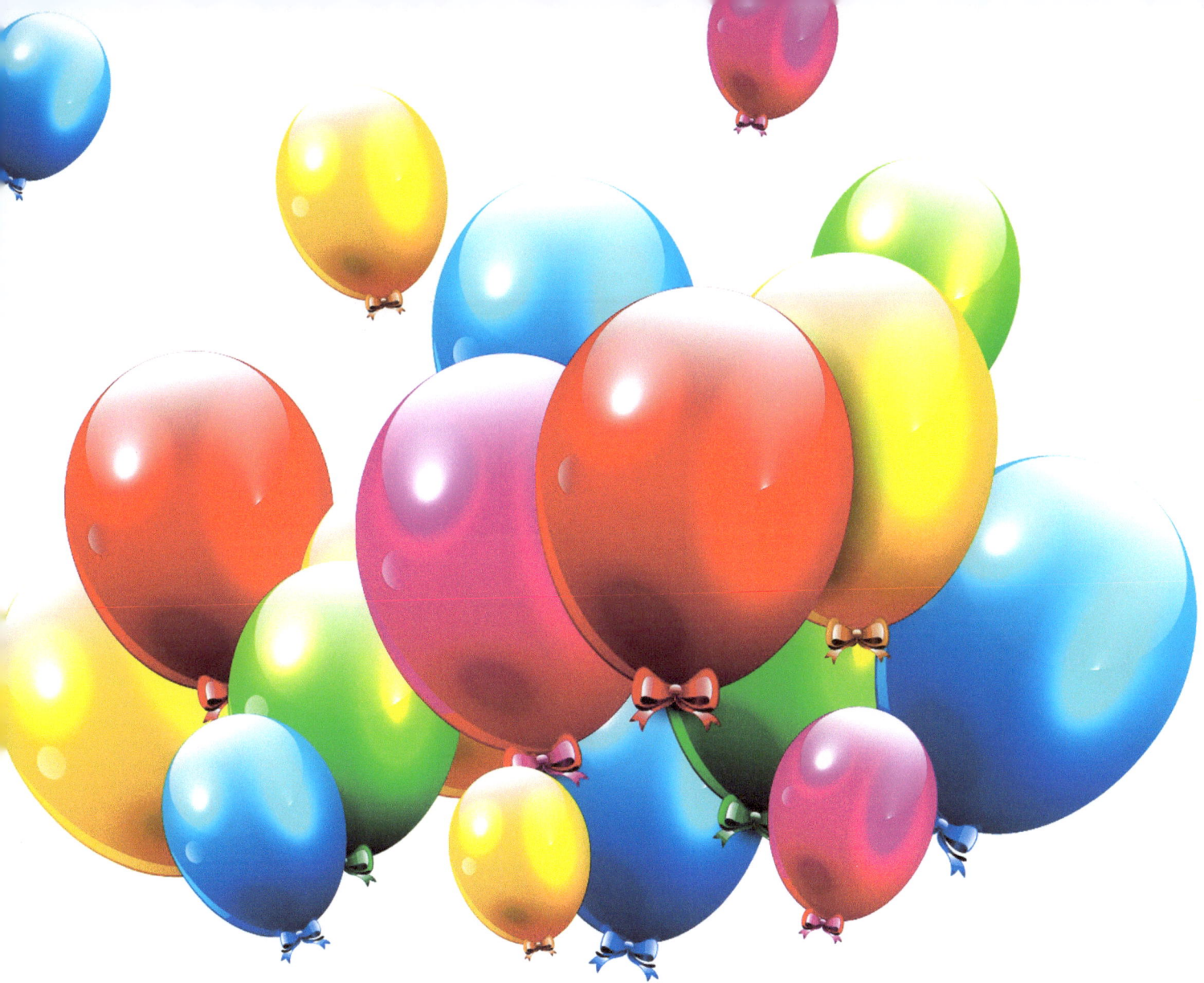

BOONU THE BALLOON SELLER – PART 2

One day, Boonu, the balloon seller, was selling balloons as usual. He sold his balloons to children as well as grownups.

While he was selling balloons, he saw the sparrow that helped him the other day. She had come to meet him.

Boonu stopped selling balloons and ran to the sparrow… the sparrow flew to Boonu…

They were very happy to meet each other.

Boonu took the sparrow to his home and gave her food and water. He also played with her. Boonu and the sparrow had a lot of fun times together.

Time passed by, and one day, the sparrow said to Boonu, "Dear friend, thank you for giving me food and water, but now I have to leave because I miss my family."

Boonu said, "Dear friend, I will let you go, but please go tomorrow because it is very dark now."

The sparrow agreed and stayed the night.

Soon, it was morning. The sparrow left. Boonu sadly left to sell balloons.

The next day when Boonu was selling balloons, he saw the sparrow again. She was flying very fast, and she was very scared...

Boonu asked her, "Why are you so scared?"

She said, "An eagle is chasing me, and that's why I am scared."

Boonu also became very scared that the eagle might harm the sparrow. He quickly took the sparrow to his home and closed the door and the windows.

But, the eagle had followed them…

The strong eagle broke a window and entered inside…

Boonu had known that the eagle would break the window and come inside. So, Boonu had already hidden the sparrow in his wardrobe.

The eagle searched and searched everywhere but could not find the sparrow. The eagle thought, 'I must have come to the wrong house.'

So, the eagle flew away.

Thus, Boonu saved the sparrow from the eagle.

Moral: Help others when they need your help, so that others will help you when you need their help.

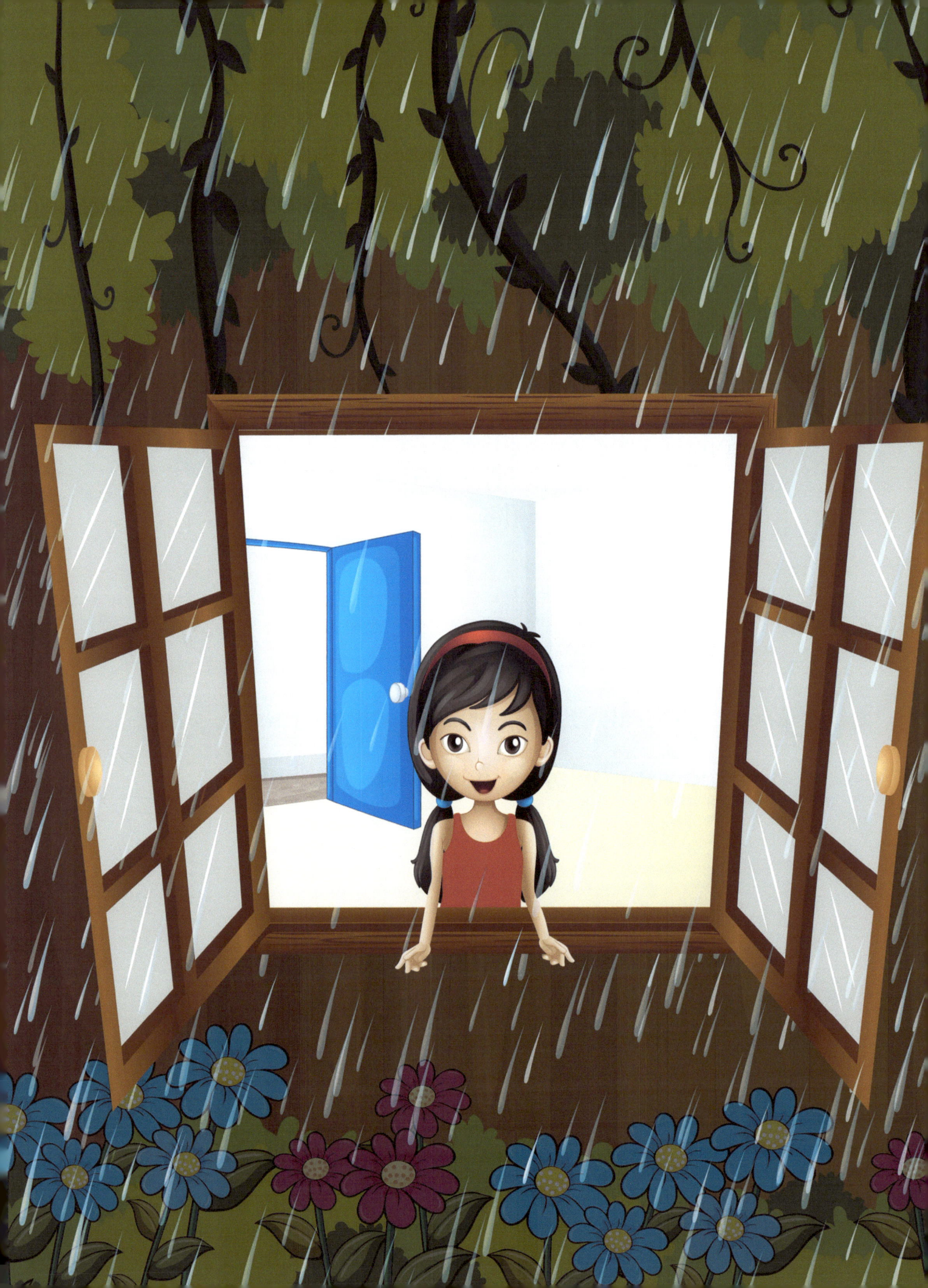

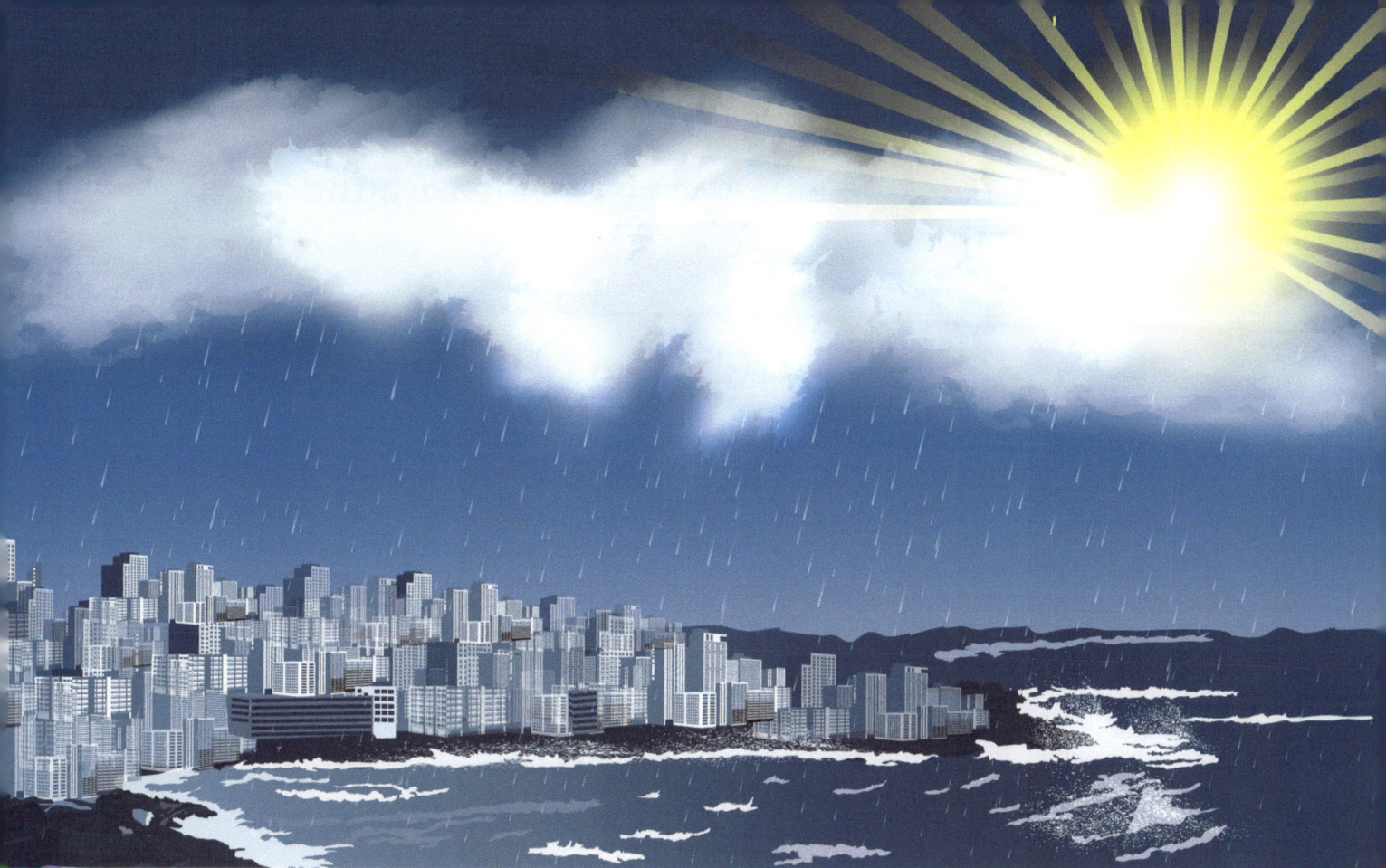

THE RAINY DAY

Once upon a time, there were two siblings, named Anoushka and Paavni. Anoushka was the elder girl, and she was in grade III, while Paavni was in KG II.

They always played together with their dolls named; Meenu, Moxie, Radha, Elsa, Anna, and Anga.

On their bed, they had built a big toy village for their dolls; it contained a restaurant, many small shops and a school and many houses.

One day, while they were playing with their dolls, it started to rain.

Anoushka and Paavni could hear the pitter patter of the rain drops on their roof.

It rained so heavily that lightening appeared like flashlights in the dark skies…

The sound of the thunder was scary…

That day it rained very heavily.

Anoushka and Paavni took their dolls downstairs, to play with. When it was time for Anoushka and Paavni to have lunch, it was still raining very heavily.

They became very scared, but they also enjoyed seeing the rain, especially Paavni.

Paavni opened a window slightly and held her hands out to the rain… rain drops fell on her hands, and it made her very happy.

Anoushka and Paavni were fascinated by the way tall trees swayed with the winds that came along with the rain.

They saw birds flying away to safe hiding places…

They were surprised to see the sky light up with lightning…

The two siblings closed their ears because the sound of the thunder was so loud…

It was a bit scary, but it was fun seeing the rain.

Moral: Learn to admire the beauty of Mother Nature and find joy in your surroundings.

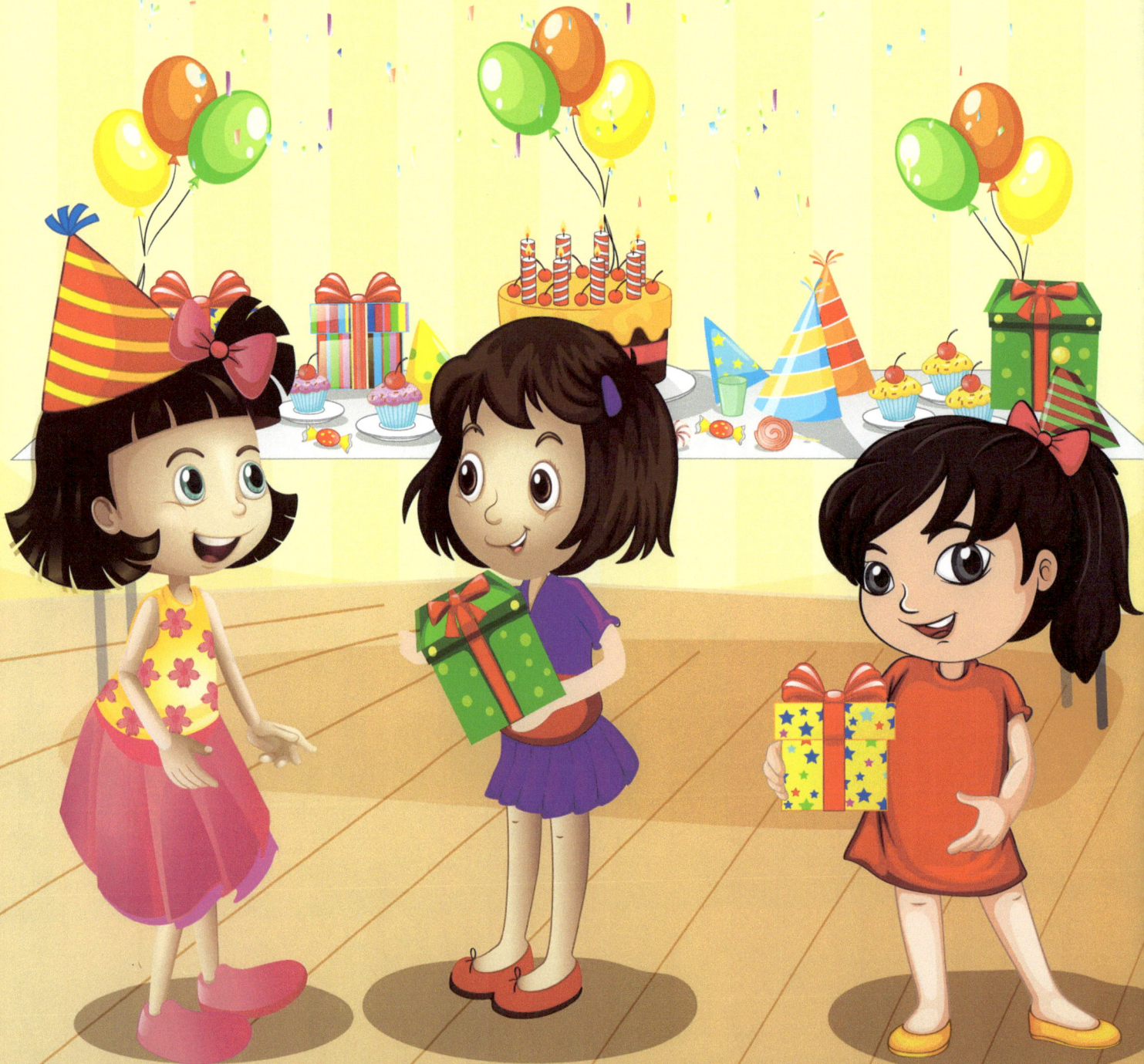

HAPPY BIRTHDAY TO SINA

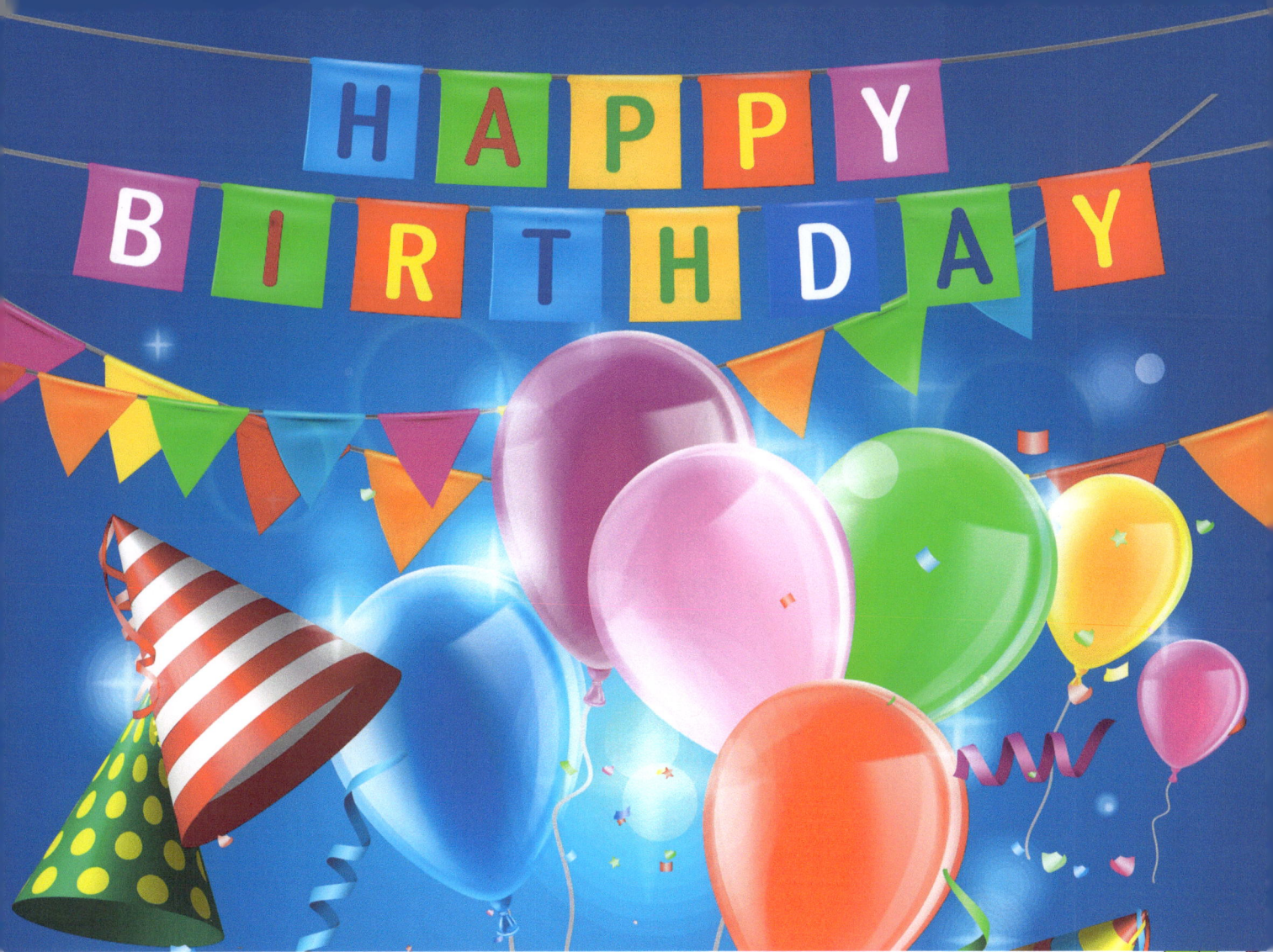

SINA'S EIGHTH BIRTHDAY

Sina was turning eight years, and her parents were arranging a birthday party for her. They sent out invitations to all her friends, family, and relatives.

On the day of her birthday party, Sina asked her mother, "At what time will everybody come to my party?"

Her mother said, "At six in the evening."

It was five in the evening. Sina got into her pink and yellow party dress. She put on pink shoes and placed a ribbon over her hair.

Soon, it was six in the evening. Her friends, family, and relatives arrived. They brought lots of gifts for Sina.

The party started, and everybody was having a great time. There were many games for children as well as parents.

Sina was happily playing with her friend Tina. Suddenly, Minnie came and pushed Tina. Tina fell down and started to cry.

Tina's friends called her parents. They said, "It will be all right. Now, stop crying and play with your friends."

Tina went back to playing with her friends. They played a lot of games like hide and seek, wall catcher etc.

Moral: Never hurt others.

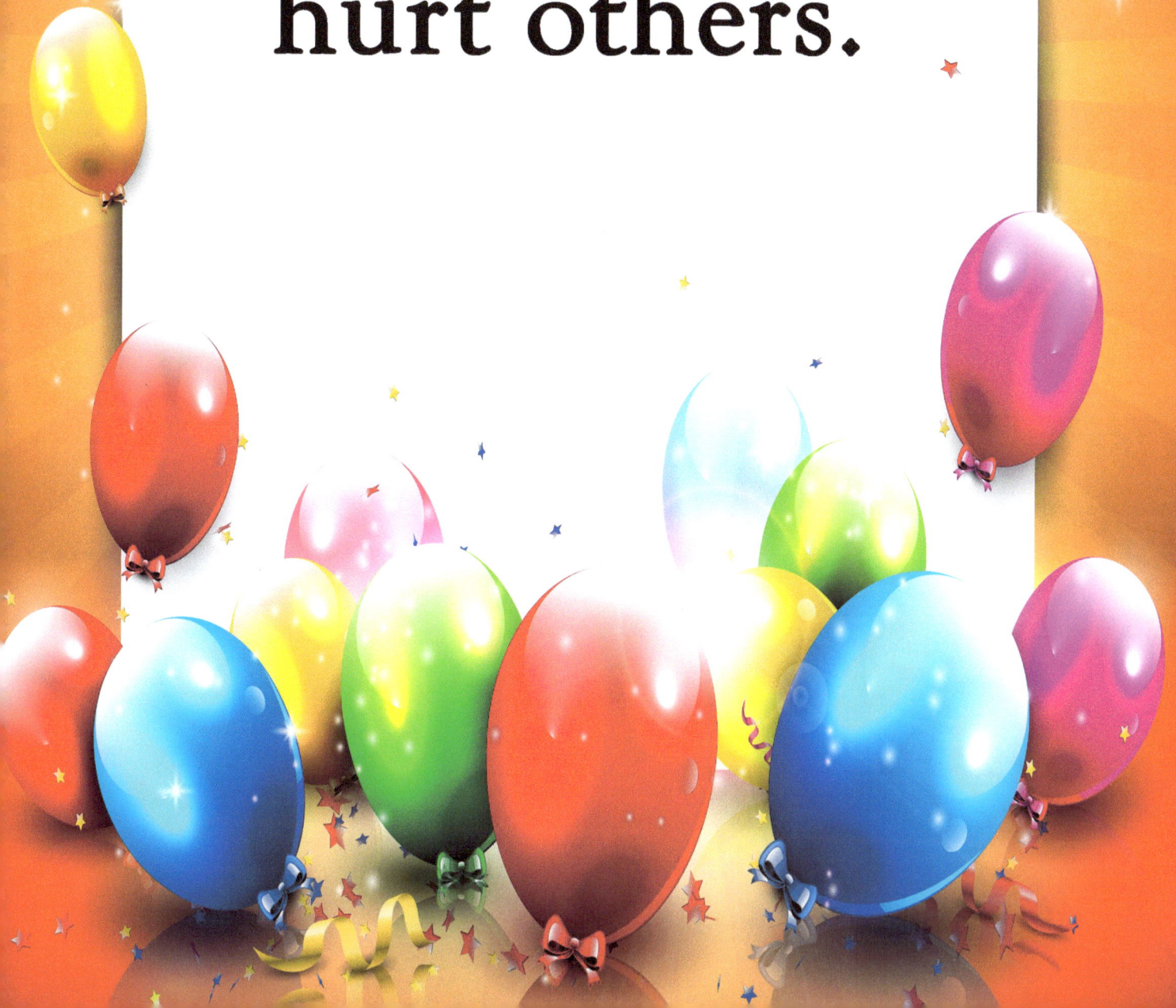

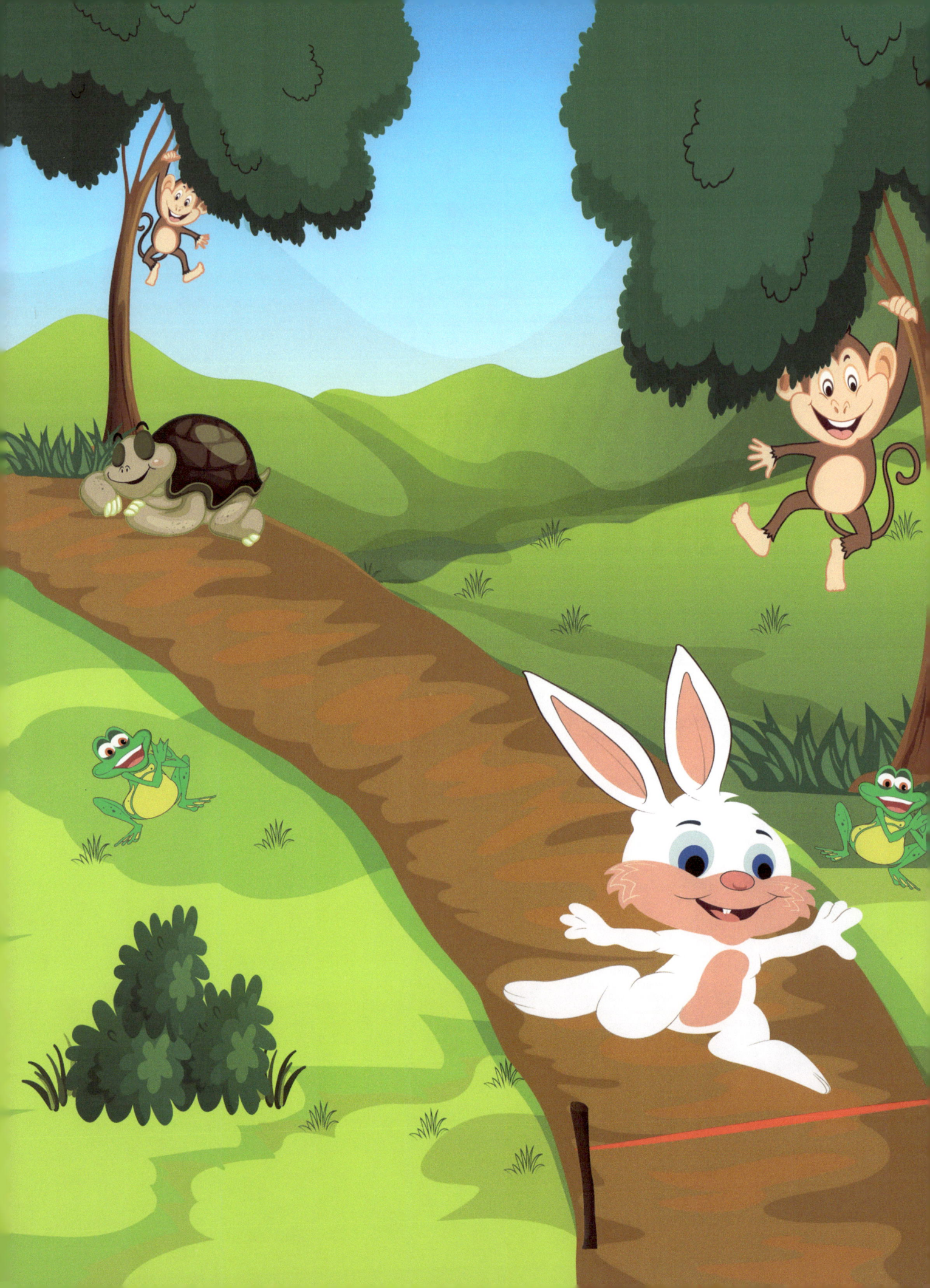

THE SLOWEST RABBIT WINS THE RACE

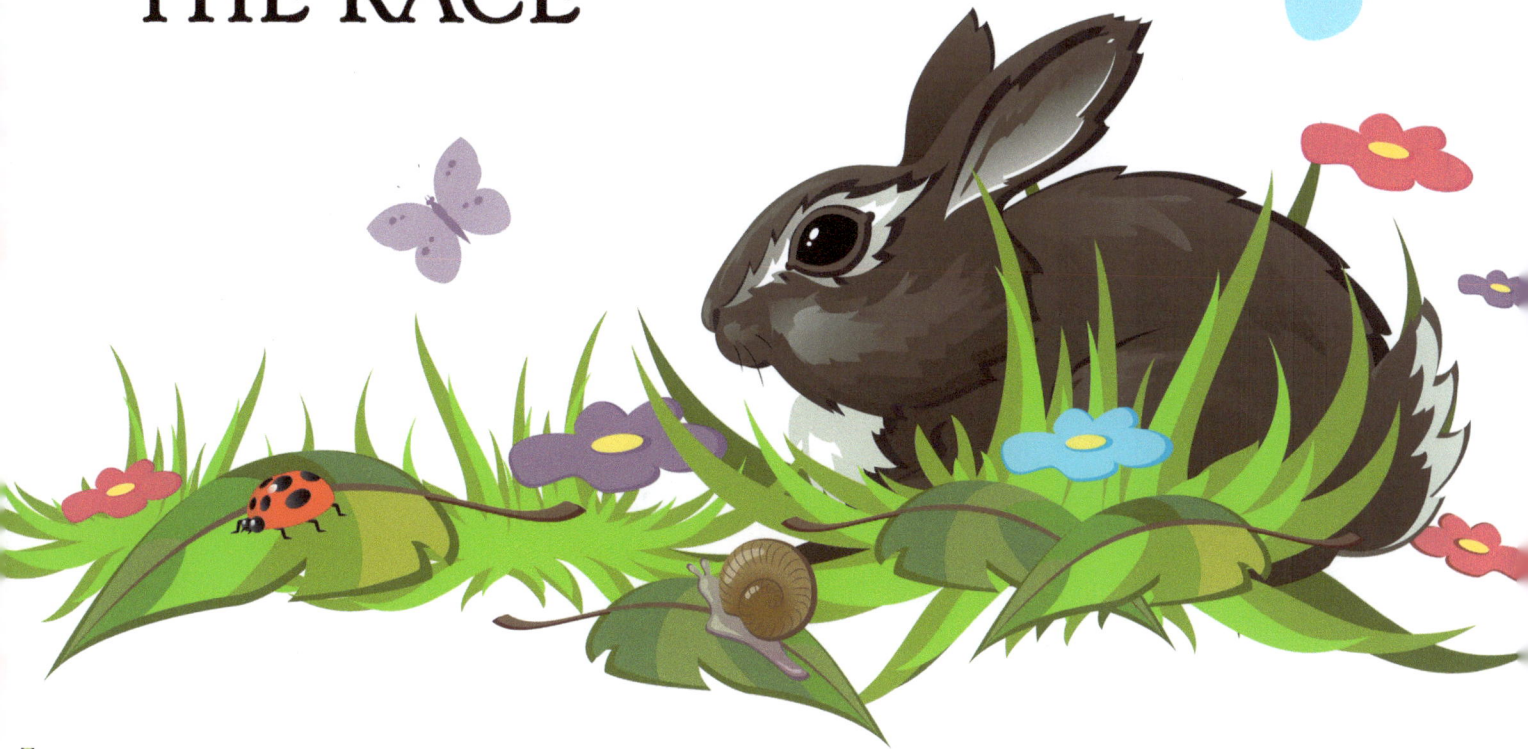

Once upon a time, there lived a very cute rabbit in a big forest.

There was something unusual about this rabbit...he couldn't run fast. Instead, he was very slow. He was slower than even a tortoise!

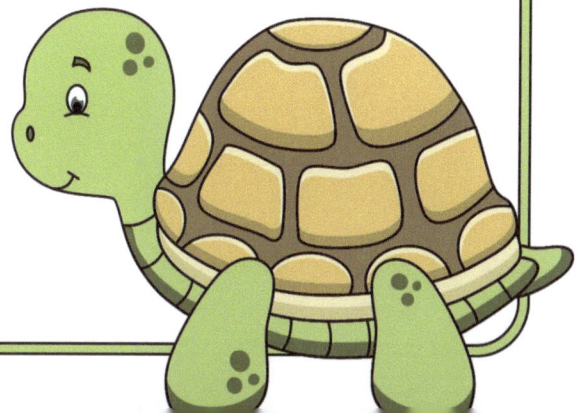

One day, a tortoise happened to see the slow rabbit. The tortoise smiled to himself thinking, 'Oh, it would be so much fun to hold a race with this slow rabbit.'

So, the tortoise said to the rabbit, "Hey rabbit, let's hold a race."

The rabbit thought about it for a while. He knew he was very slow – slower than even the tortoise. But the rabbit agreed to race with the tortoise.

The tortoise said, "Let's race tomorrow at five in the evening."

Soon, it dawned to tomorrow.

The tortoise was very certain that he was going to win the race.

As the race started, the rabbit began to walk very slowly.

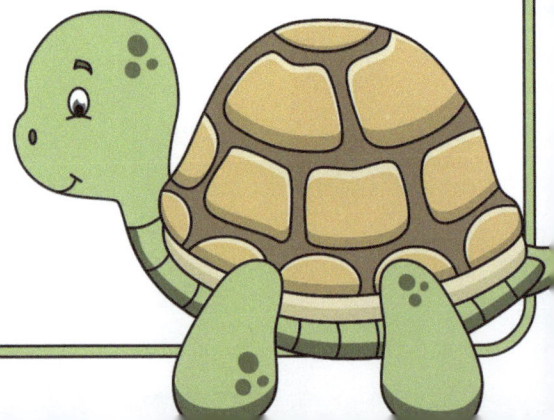

The tortoise looked back and saw that the rabbit was walking very slowly. The tortoise thought, 'Let me take a rest for some time. The rabbit is very slow, and there is no way he could keep up with me.'

So, the tortoise slept cozily under a shady tree.

When the rabbit reached where the tortoise was sleeping, the rabbit passed by very slowly, without making any sound.

The rabbit continued to walk and walk...and finally; he reached the finish line.

Suddenly, the tortoise woke up. He thought, 'I must start walking to the finish line.'

But when the tortoise approached the finish line, he was surprised to see that the rabbit had already reached the finish line before him.

Thus, the very slow rabbit won the race!

The tortoise was very sad.

The rabbit was very happy.

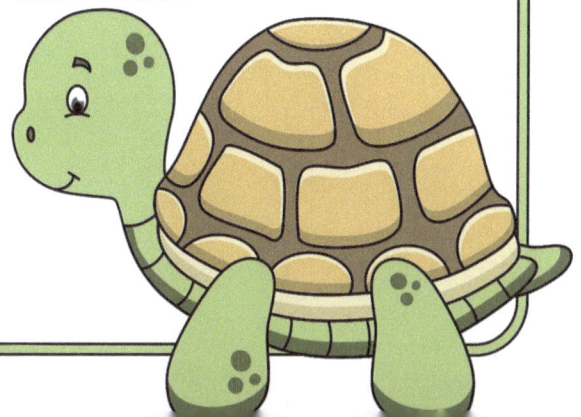

Moral: Slow and steady wins the race.

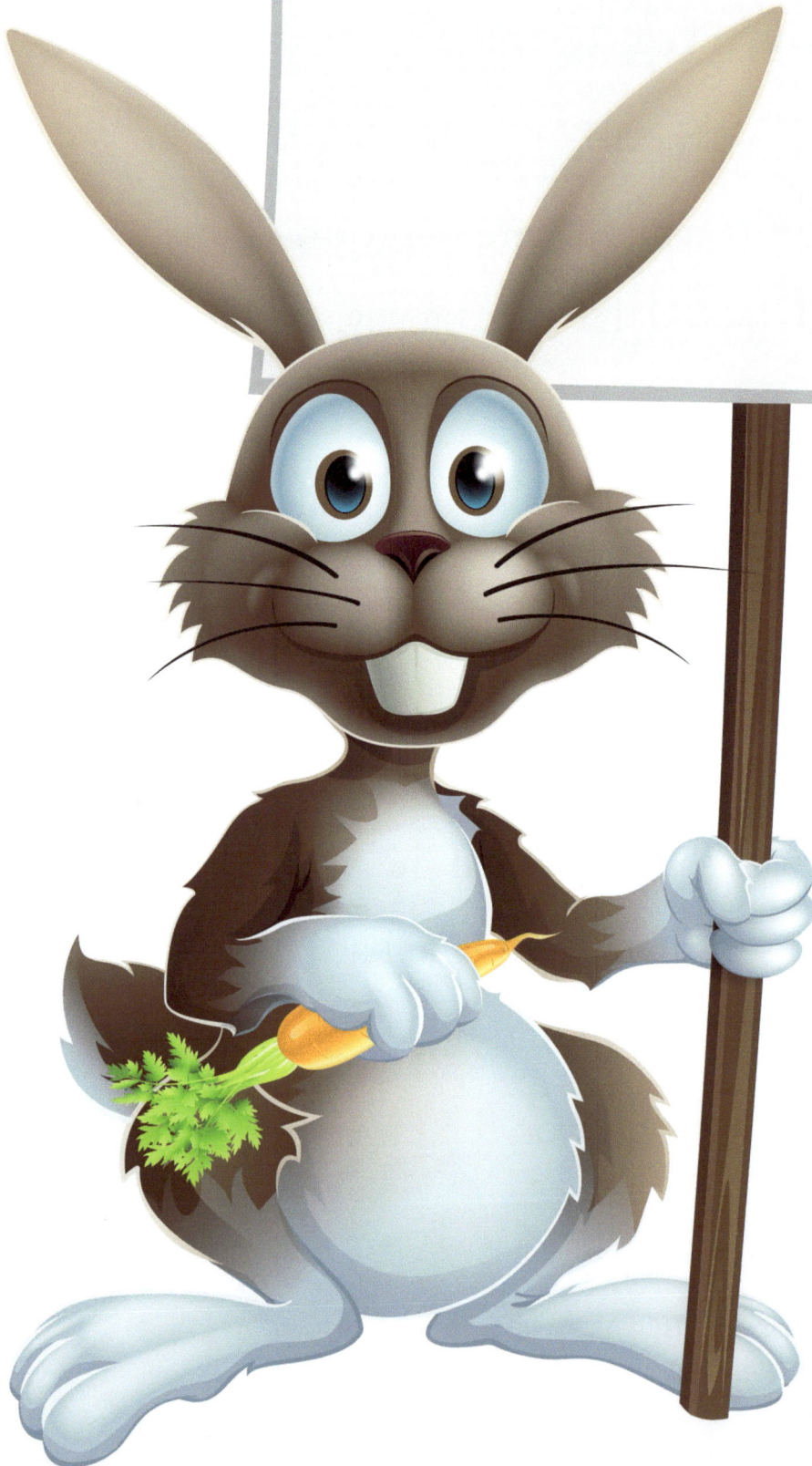